Exercises
for Joints & Glands

Exercises
for Joints & Glands

Simple Movements to Enhance Your Well-Being

AS TAUGHT BY SWAMI RAMA

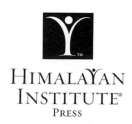

HIMALAYAN
INSTITUTE®
PRESS

Himalayan Institute Press
952 Bethany Turnpike
Honesdale, PA 18431

www.HimalayanInstitute.org

First edition 1977
Second edition 2007

ISBN-13: 978-0-89389-264-7
ISBN-10:   0-89389-264-5

Printed in Thailand

Photography by Jagati

The paper used in this publication meets the minimum requirements of American National Standard for Information Sciences—Permanence of Paper for Printed Library Materials,
ANSI Z39.48-1984.

Library of Congress Cataloging-in-Publication Data

Rama, Swami, 1925-
  Exercises for joints and glands : simple movements to enhance your well-being / as taught by Swami Rama. -- 2nd ed.
      p. cm.
  ISBN-13: 978-0-89389-264-7 (alk. paper)
  ISBN-10: 0-89389-264-5 (alk. paper)
  1. Hatha yoga. 2. Joints. 3. Glands. I. Title.
  RA781.7.R263 2007
  613.7'046--dc22
                                                    2007020647

One of the greatest adepts, teachers, writers, and humanitarians of the 20th century, Swami Rama is the founder of the Himalayan Institute. Born in northern India, he was raised from early childhood by a Himalayan sage, Bengali Baba. Under the guidance of his master he traveled from monastery to monastery and studied with a variety of Himalayan saints and sages, including his grandmaster, who lived in a remote region of Tibet. In addition to this intense spiritual training, Swami Rama received higher education in both India and Europe. From 1949 to 1952, he held the prestigious position of Shankaracharya of Karvirpitham in south India. Thereafter, he returned to his master to receive further training at his cave monastery, and in 1969 came to the United States where he founded the Himalayan Institute. His best known work, *Living with the Himalayan Masters,* reveals the many facets of this exceptional adept and demonstrates his embodiment of the living tradition of the East.

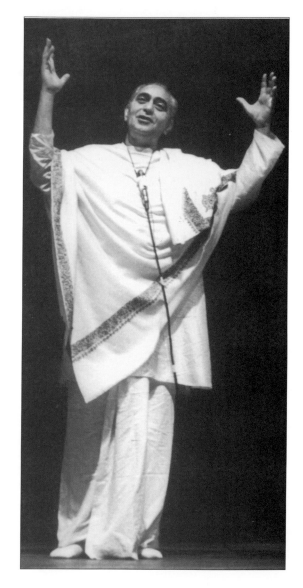

Table of Contents

FOREWORD   ix
INTRODUCTION   xi
GENERAL INSTRUCTIONS   xiii

SEATED EXERCISES   1–21
- Preparation   2
- Face
  Forehead and Sinus Massage   4
  Scalp and Forehead Squeeze   6
  Half-Face Squint   6
  Full-Face Squint   7
- Eyes
  Guidelines   8
  Peripheral Stretch   8
  Eye Angles   10
  Eye Circles   12
  Eye Focus   13
- Mouth & Full Face
  Mouth Stretches   14
  Lion Pose   16
  Face Massage   17
- Neck
  Neck Stretches   18
  Chin Over Shoulder   19
  Ear Over Shoulder   19
  Turtle   20
  Neck Rolls   21

STANDING EXERCISES   23–53
- Preparation   24
- Shoulders
  Shoulder Shrugs   25
  Rotations with
    Relaxed Arms   26
  Vertical Arm Swings   28
  Horizontal Arm Swings   29
  Rotations with Extended Arms   30
  Chest Expander   32
  Shoulder Wings   34
  Arm Circles   35

■ Hands & Wrists
   Wrist Bends   36
   Hand Circles   38

■ Abdomen & Torso
   Horizontal Arm Stretch   40
   Overhead Stretch   41
   Standing Side Bend   42
   Supported Torso Rotation   43
   Abdominal Squeeze   44
   Forward Stretch   45

■ Legs & Feet
   Leg Swings   46
   Leg Kicks   47
   Knee Swirls   48
   Dancing Knees   49
   Ankle Exercises   50
   Foot Circles   52
   Toe Balance   53

HANDS & KNEES EXERCISES 55–61
■ Preparation   56
■ Torso & Pelvis
   Cat Pose   57
   Cat Pose Twist   58
   Lunge Pose   59
   Boat Pose   60
   Simple Seated Twist   61

FLOOR EXERCISES   63–69
■ Preparation   64
■ Pelvis & Legs
   Knees to Chest Pose   65
   Reclining Leg Cradles   66
   Pelvic Tilt   67

■ Systematic Relaxation in
   Corpse Pose   68

ABBREVIATED SEQUENCE   71–75

Foreword

If you watch a cat or a dog when it wakes up, you'll see that it goes through an elaborate process of stretching. One leg, for example, is put far back and the body is stretched away from it as much as possible. You may do something similar when you climb out of bed in the morning. Putting your arms high above your head and stretching up from the tips of your toes seems like a natural part of coming out of sleep.

But why do you do this? Mostly because it feels good. You may not think about it much, but it seems to get the body back into comfortable working order. It re-coordinates the system and makes you feel more alive.

At first glance it seems like an insignificant thing, this luxurious morning stretch. But there is a very important underlying principle. Researchers have begun to discover the importance of what they call the body image. Our mental picture of ourselves determines to a great extent which parts of our body we use actively and which parts we tend to forget. A person whose awareness centers around his face and chest, for instance, may have a pleasant expression and dress neatly, while he tends to ignore his spine and the back part of his body. His basic posture suffers as a result. He will, without being particularly conscious of it, allow his upper spine to slump into a hunchback position. After years of habitually sitting and standing this way, the back becomes "frozen." In a sense it doesn't get the energy that is necessary to keep it flexible and healthy. Calcifications and other disorders of the spine are likely to follow.

We might say, then, that when we forget a part of our body, it suffers serious consequences. When it is not properly positioned, movements around it are not properly regulated. One set of muscles becomes weak from disuse, another over-developed from the effort to maintain an off-balance position.

Yoga postures are designed to break up such bad habits by systematically exercising different parts of the body in a gentle, pleasant way. We can gradually bring back into our awareness muscles and joints that have been forgotten over the years. Muscles that had become weak are gradually and gently strengthened so that the body can once more be held in a comfortable and natural position. Posture is improved so that energy may begin to flow again in a natural, exhilarating way.

In yoga, the basis for these exercises is outlined in great detail. The physical body is said to be only one of several bodies that make up the human system. The way we picture ourselves, our mental image of our shape, is part of what is called the mental body. Besides this and the physical body that we can see and touch, there is an intermediate level that has to do with the energy that activates our muscles, glands, and so forth. We might compare it to the electricity that makes a motor run. The energy must flow through the right channels and enter the right circuits if the machine is to function smoothly. The energy, the physical body, and the mental body image interact in an intricate way. But we do not need to trouble ourselves with the theory in order to enjoy the benefits of yogic exercises.

In fact, it is not even necessary to struggle with the complex and difficult poses that are usually described in yoga manuals. Actually, they only become really useful once the body has begun to move back toward a natural balance. Meanwhile, the joint and gland exercises are a set of simple, pleasant stretches that can be used with great benefit by almost anyone, regardless of how badly out of shape they are. By increasing the circulation to different parts of the body and by restoring a natural, flowing body image in the mind, a harmonious feeling of energy throughout the system can be re-established. This means that all the structures, including the joints and glands, benefit. One beneficial effect of the exercises accentuates another. The results can be very gratifying. It comes as a surprise to many people that they can feel better each day instead of worse!

It should be kept in mind that these are stretches. They should be as pleasant and enjoyable as that first exuberant stretch that comes spontaneously on stepping out of bed. Done slowly, gently, and with enjoyment, they can be most effective.

Rudolph M. Ballentine, MD

Introduction ■

Swami Rama, the teacher of the joints and glands exercises found in this book, is one of the giant figures in the development of yoga in the West. After his arrival in the United States in 1969, he traveled tirelessly, highlighting the need for an introspective view of life, inspiring students, and giving special attention to the various practices of yoga and meditation. In 1970, he visited the Menninger Foundation in Topeka, Kansas, where he demonstrated self-regulation abilities that changed the course of Western research and that remain, to this day, unmatched feats of inner and outer control. Not long after, he founded the Himalayan International Institute, a vehicle for educational and charitable work with a global outreach. The Institute's headquarters in Honesdale, Pennsylvania, continues to act as a center for the development of this work under the guidance of Pandit Rajmani Tigunait.

As a teacher, Swami Rama minimized the mystical expectations students projected on him. "Do not try to leap ahead!" he would remind his audiences. "Tread the path systematically. Practice faithfully and let your life unfold in its own time." Thus, from the earliest days, he carefully developed instruction that could be embraced by students at all levels—instruction that often proved deceptively beneficial.

The exercises found here are among the very first techniques he taught. He recommended that all students practice these exercises for at least four weeks prior to beginning more demanding asanas. In the process, he said, students would reconnect with their bodies, develop balance and flexibility, improve their posture, and learn to coordinate movements with breathing. Since these exercises are not athletically challenging and require only moderate strength, they are suitable for virtually all students.

These exercises can be used for long-term practice as well. They maintain supple joints and enhance a general sense of well-being, qualities that are particularly important as the body ages. The exercises are also highly recommended for persons suffering from arthritis, rheumatism, and habitual stiffness. They offer a safe way to get started toward better health.

The exercises are sequenced to begin in a sitting posture and work down through the body, from head to toes. In some cases, massage is combined with the exercises. A central goal is to stimulate blood flow to each area of the body, flushing out wastes and toxins, and supplying the body with fresh nutrients.

Loss of health and mobility begins with such impediments as stiff ankles, sore shoulder joints, tension around the eyes and face, a rigid spinal column, and tightness in the wrists and finger joints. In addition, soreness in the lower back and rigidity in the hip joints are extraordinarily common ailments. It is surprising how effectively these problems can be addressed with repetitions of the relatively simple movements found here.

The exercises also benefit the mind and nervous system. As the body becomes more calm and relaxed, a natural sense of peacefulness arises. Concentration improves and there is a lightness to being in one's body that makes everyday movements easier. Hormone-secreting glands that play an integral role in the process of stress and nervous system arousal are regulated and pacified. And the sequence concludes with systematic relaxation, a deeply calming experience for body and mind.

Swami Rama was concerned that beginning students of every age and qualification receive well-balanced instruction. Once, many years ago in Nepal, an elderly couple joined him for lunch, where they spoke animatedly about many subjects. Afterward the couple asked whether Swami Rama was willing to give them something to practice in their daily life. He taught them several exercises from this book, including the abdominal squeeze. After the couple left he wondered aloud whether I knew them. I was certain I did not. "He is the Chief Justice of the Supreme Court," Swami Rama said casually.

Rolf Sovik, PsyD

General Instructions ■

To receive the greatest benefits from the exercises in this book, practice regularly, move slowly, and concentrate on your movements. Be sure to practice on an empty stomach and bladder; two hours after a light meal or four hours after a heavy meal is recommended. Maintain an awareness of your breath at all times, and, unless otherwise specified, breathe through your nose.

Precautions: Many physical problems benefit from the appropriate practice of yoga, but please check with your health-care professional and work with a well-trained teacher if you have serious health problems. This manual is not intended to replace personal instruction or professional medical advice. The contraindications listed for some exercises are guidelines only. If you have abnormal blood pressure, a back injury, or any other serious health problem, or if you have had surgery recently, please consult your physician before beginning your practice.

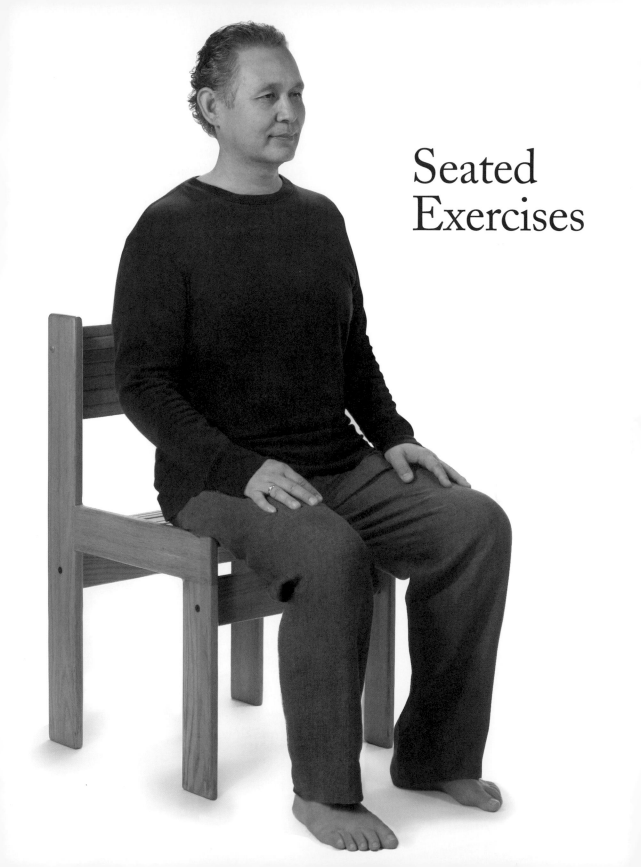

Seated
Exercises

■ Preparation

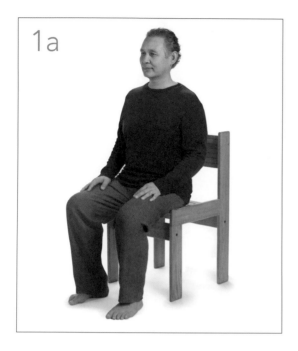

1a

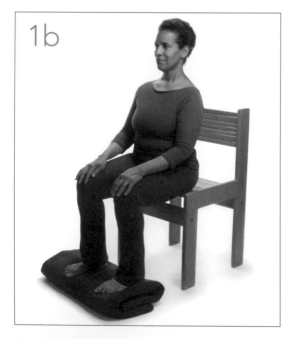

1b

Begin by sitting comfortably on a chair with a firm, flat surface. Place your feet flat on the floor and parallel to one another *(fig. 1a)*. For comfort, your thighs should slope slightly down toward your knees, with your ankles aligned directly beneath your knees. If the chair is too high, place folded blankets under your feet to achieve the proper angle for your legs *(fig. 1b)*. If the chair is too low, place the folded blankets on the seat to raise your hips.

If you are able, you may sit cross-legged on the floor instead. If you choose to sit on the floor, place your legs in a comfortable cross-legged position. Sit on the edge of a cushion or a stack of folded blankets so that your hips are slightly higher than your knees *(fig. 2)*. With your sit bones well grounded, elevate through your lower back and lift your rib cage slightly. Relax your shoulders to the sides, so they are neither forward nor back. Rest your hands softly on your thighs. Elongate the back of your neck, drawing the head back and lengthening through the crown.

When your body is aligned in this way, your muscles do not have to work hard to hold you in place, and they can soften and relax. Come back to this simple posture after each of the exercises in the seated sequence and rest for a moment, being aware of how you feel in your body. Notice each time if and how the exercises have changed how you feel.

Before you begin the following exercises, take a moment to be aware of your breathing. Close your eyes and feel your breath flowing in and out for a few breaths. Without changing your alignment, soften your abdomen and the sides of your rib cage, so they can expand and contract effortlessly with each breath. Observe the different sensations on inhalation and exhalation, and, by doing so, feel your breath become smooth, deep, and even. Maintain this awareness throughout the exercises and as you rest between them.

Unless otherwise indicated, repeat each exercise 3 times, but avoid going beyond your capacity. If you feel strain, stop and relax, then proceed more gently. These exercises should feel good.

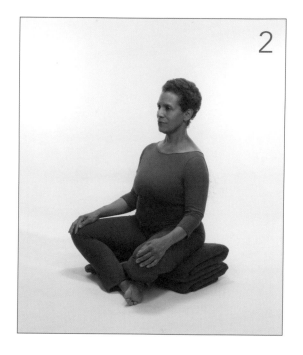

2

■ Face

Forehead and Sinus Massage

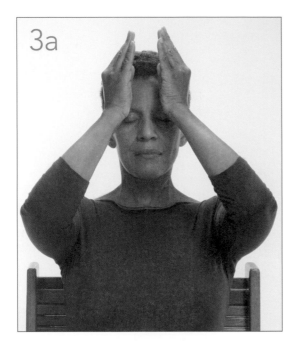

The movements in this sequence begin at the center of the face and move outward, drawing tensions away from the face, forehead, and temples, and smoothing wrinkles on the forehead and around the corners of the eyes. This massage may also help loosen mucus obstructions in the nasal sinuses.

Place the tip of each thumb at the base of the small finger. This will expose the soft, fleshy portion of the thumb to use for massage. Now place this fleshy base of the thumb against your forehead between your eyebrows *(fig. 3a)*.

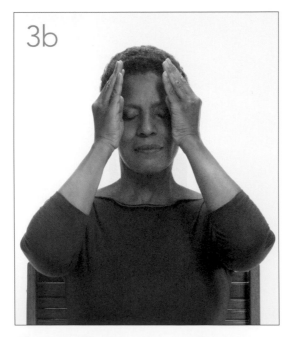

Massage your forehead by drawing your thumbs up and out with a stroking motion. Using gentle pressure, follow the bony structure around your eyes, and continue out toward the temples. Using the same hand position, place your thumbs just below your eyes along each side of the bridge of your nose. Draw the fleshy part of your thumbs along your cheekbones out toward the temples *(fig. 3b)*.

Next, open your hands. Use the thumb and index finger of each hand to squeeze and knead your eyebrows from the center toward the temples. Imagine that you are kneading small lumps of dough *(fig. 4a)*. Repeat the movement a number of times, but be sure not to press on the eyeballs themselves.

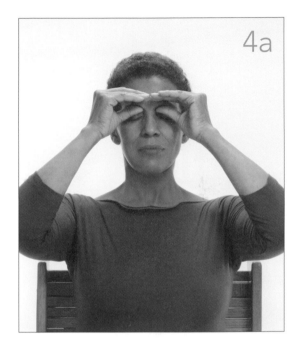

Next, using the fleshy undersides of your index fingers, massage the lower rim of your eye sockets, working along the cheekbone from the sides of the nose toward the temples *(fig. 4b)*. Again, take care not to press directly on the eyeballs themselves.

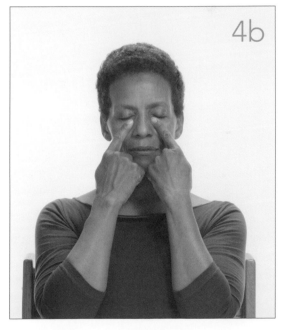

◼ Face

Scalp and Forehead Squeeze

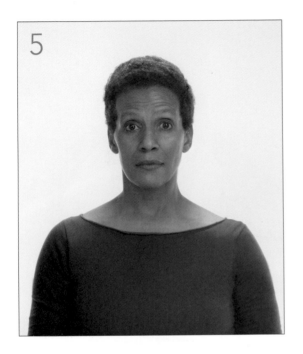

Keep your eyes focused straight ahead and your head stationary. Inhale, and with a smooth movement, lift your eyebrows and forehead as high as you can. Create tension and wrinkles in your forehead *(fig. 5)*.

As you exhale, slowly lower your eyebrows, releasing the tension from the forehead and softening the muscles completely.

Half-Face Squint

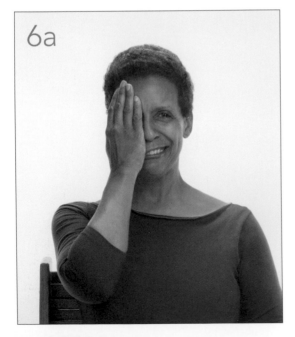

Place your right hand gently over the right side of your face. This side of your face will remain completely relaxed throughout the following exercise. Now, squint with the entire left side of your face, firmly contracting the muscles to create tension *(fig. 6a)*. Continue breathing as you hold the tension. Then relax, releasing the tension from your face and softening the muscles completely.

Repeat the squint on the right side *(fig. 6b)*. The division between the muscles tensed and the muscles relaxed should be definite. One eye should be tense and the other relaxed. Half the mouth should be tense and half relaxed. When you are comfortable with this exercise, you can do it without using your hands.

Repeat twice more on each side. Then relax.

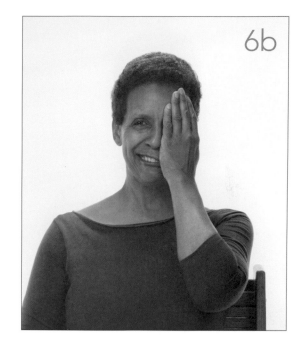

Full-Face Squint

Squeeze your eyes shut, wrinkle your nose, purse your lips, and tense all the muscles of your face, pulling them toward the tip of your nose, as if your nose were the center of gravity *(fig. 7)*. Continue to breathe as you hold the tension. Then relax, softening the muscles completely. Repeat twice more.

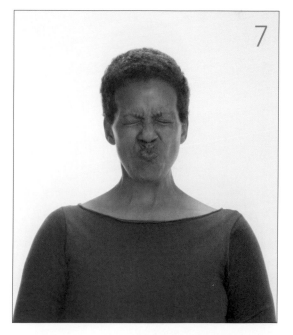

■ Eyes

Guidelines

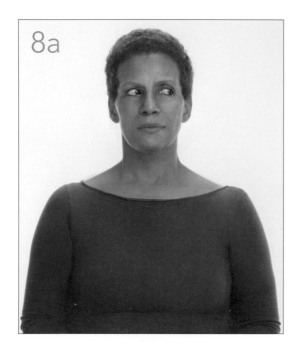

Keep your head stationary and your facial muscles relaxed throughout the following eye exercises. If you hold any of the movements, be sure to hold for the same length of time in each direction, maintaining a relaxed and even flow of breath throughout. After some practice, all the eye movements can be coordinated with breathing—exhaling in one direction and inhaling in the other (or vice versa). After each variation, relax your eyes by gently closing them for several seconds.

Peripheral Stretch

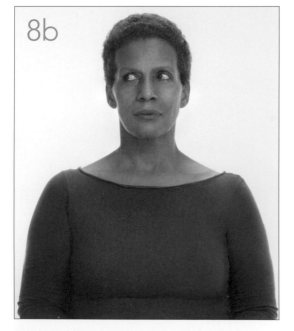

Begin by looking straight ahead. Shift your gaze to the left as if to look toward the corner of your eye. Feel the stretch in the eye muscles *(fig. 8a)*. Slowly return your gaze to the center. Then repeat to the right *(fig. 8b)*. After 3 repetitions on each side, return to the center and relax your eyes.

Again, begin by looking straight ahead. Without moving your head, lift your gaze slowly up toward the ceiling *(fig. 8c)*, and then slowly lower it back to the center.

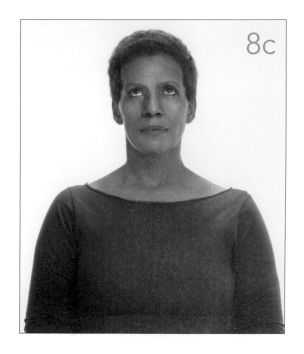

Now lower your gaze as if to look at the floor *(fig. 8d)*, and then return to the center. After 3 repetitions in each direction, rest with your eyes closed.

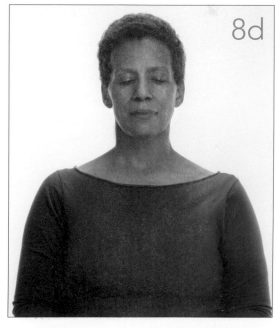

■ Eyes

Eye Angles

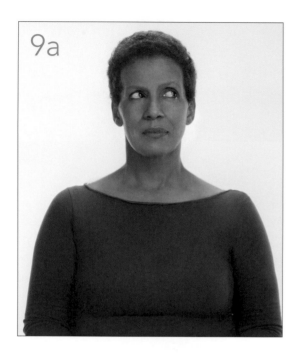

From the center, slowly shift your gaze to the upper-left-hand corner *(fig. 9a)*. Then slowly return to the center.

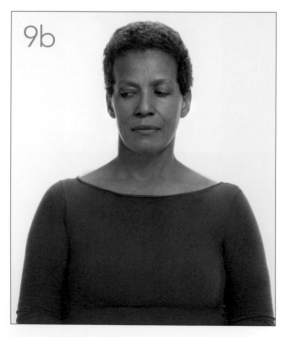

Next, look to the lower-right-hand corner *(fig. 9b)*, and then come back to the center. After 3 repetitions in each direction, rest your eyes at the center.

From the center, slowly shift your gaze to the lower-left-hand corner *(fig. 9c)*. Then return your eyes to the center.

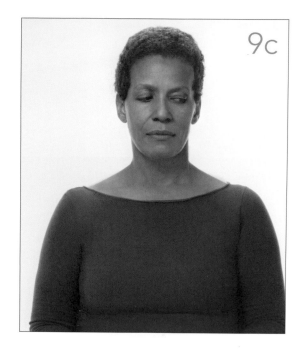

Next, look to the upper-right-hand corner *(fig. 9d)*, and then return to the center. After 3 repetitions in each direction, rest with your eyes closed.

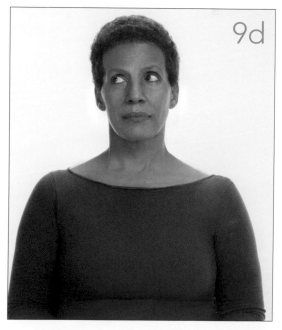

■ Eyes

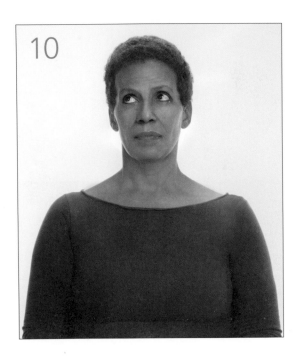

Eye Circles

Begin by lowering your gaze toward the bottom of the eye sockets. Now, circle your gaze in a clockwise direction around the entire periphery of your eyes *(fig. 10)*. Move smoothly, without jerks or pauses. After 3 repetitions, reverse the motion, circling the eyes in a counterclockwise direction. Then, close your eyes and let them rest.

Eye Focus

Lift your hand in front of your face, an arm's length away. Make a loose fist with the back of the thumb facing toward you and pointing up. Rest your gaze on the thumb *(fig. 11)*. With a smooth, gentle motion, slowly draw your hand closer to your face without averting your gaze. When your eyes begin to lose their focus, stop your hand and hold your gaze. If you are able to regain focus by relaxing, draw your hand a little closer and hold your gaze again. Repeat until you can no longer achieve a clear focus. Then smoothly draw your hand back to its starting position.

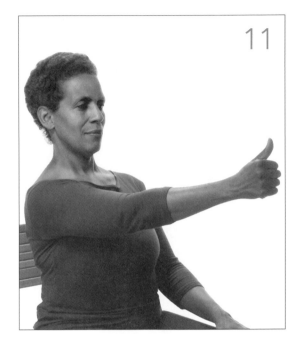

To complete the eye exercises, close your eyes and squeeze the lids together tightly for 5 seconds. Then, open your eyes and blink your eyelids as rapidly as you can for 5 seconds. Rest your eyes by closing them gently so that the eyelids only lightly touch. Hold for 5 seconds. Finally, rub the palms of your hands together rapidly to create warmth, and cup your warm palms over your closed eyes for 5 seconds or more—without pressing on the eyeballs *(fig. 12)*. Let your eyes completely relax.

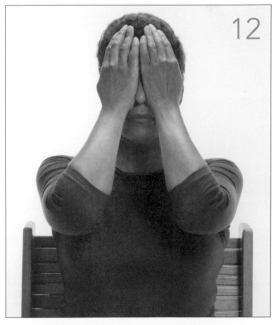

■ Mouth & Full Face

Mouth Stretches

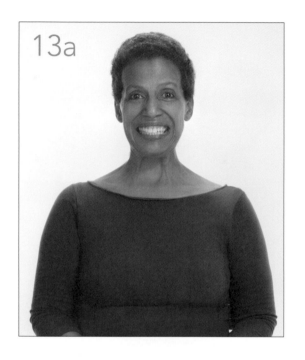

As you inhale, grit your teeth and stretch your lips in a wide grin *(fig. 13a)*. The muscles and tendons of your neck should protrude like cords stretching from underneath your chin to your shoulders. Hold for a number of breaths and then relax as you exhale, softening the muscles completely.

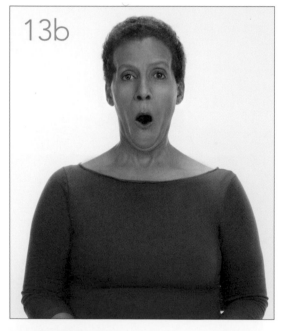

Next, open your mouth and stretch it into the shape of an O, lowering your chin and pulling your lips tightly over your teeth, so your teeth do not show. Again, hold and breathe for a number of breaths *(fig. 13b)*.

Then, keeping your mouth as far open as possible, curl the upper lip back, as if to touch the nose, and curl the lower lip down, as if to touch the chin *(fig. 13c)*.

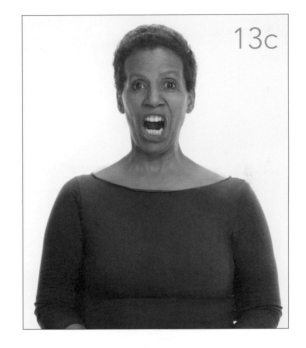

Finally, close your mouth and curl both lips up toward the tip of your nose *(fig. 13d)*. Then relax, softening the muscles around the mouth completely.

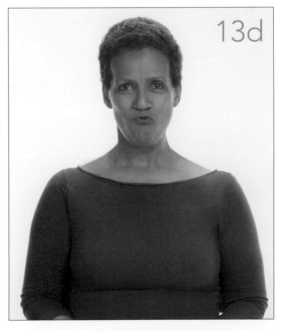

◼ Mouth & Full Face

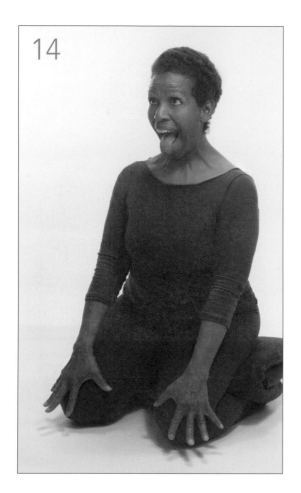

Lion Pose

This dramatic exercise stimulates circulation to the throat, relaxes the voice box, and improves sore throat, bad breath, and clarity of speech. It is also said to strengthen the intellect.

To begin, sit on the front of a chair, or kneel with your buttocks resting on the heels (for comfort you can support your buttocks or ankles with a cushion). Place your hands on your knees, palms down. Now, open your mouth as wide as possible and exhale forcefully, slightly lifting your hips and tipping forward. Thrust your tongue out and down, as if trying to touch the chin, and lift your gaze to the point between your eyebrows. Straighten your arms and extend them slightly forward with fingers spread apart as far as possible *(fig. 14)*. Your entire body is engaged in this "ferocious" posture.

Face Massage

Using the heels of your hands, massage your entire face, following the bony structures of your forehead, eyes, cheeks, jaw, mouth, and chin. Work deeply, drawing muscle, fascia, and skin away from the center of the face and out toward your temples *(fig. 15)*.

This massage removes any remaining tension in the facial muscles and smoothes out wrinkles resulting from tension in the face.

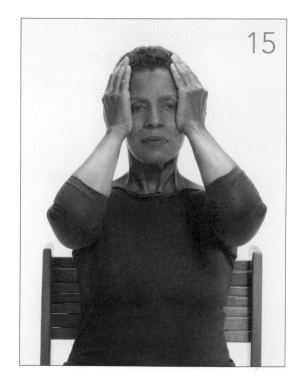

■ Neck

Neck Stretches

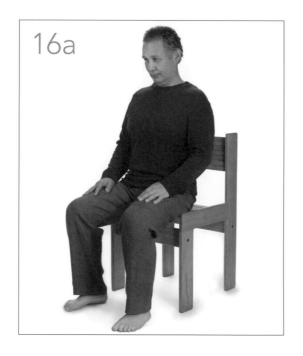

In the following neck exercises, your shoulders remain still. Only your neck and head move.

Sit with your head, neck, and trunk erect. As you exhale, retract your head (like a turtle), and tuck your chin toward your chest to elongate the back of your neck *(fig. 16a)*.

Feel the stretch along the muscles in the back of the neck, extending down into the upper back.

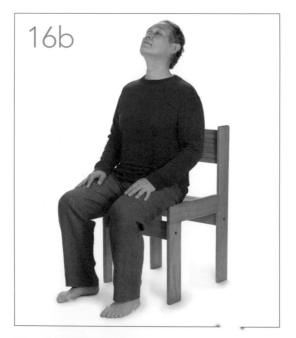

As you inhale, lift your head to the starting position, lengthen the back of the neck, and reach your chin upward, stretching the muscles along the front of your neck and top of your chest *(fig. 16b)*. Exhaling, lower the head and continue until you have completed 3 repetitions. Then return to the starting position.

Chin Over Shoulder

Sit erect. As you exhale, twist your neck to the left, keeping your chin parallel to the floor *(fig. 16c)*. Turn as far as comfortable, drawing your chin toward your shoulder. As you inhale, return your head to the starting position. Repeat on the right side. Then continue twice more on each side.

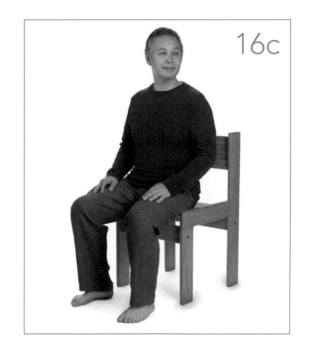

16c

Ear Over Shoulder

Sit erect. As you exhale, tip your neck to the left and lower your left ear toward your left shoulder *(fig. 16d)*. Be sure to keep your shoulders relaxed and still. Do not raise the shoulder to meet the ear. As you inhale, raise your head to the starting position. Repeat on the right side. Then continue twice more on each side.

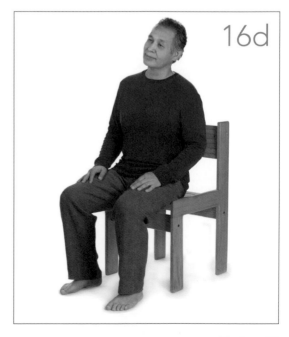

16d

■ Neck

Turtle

Sit erect. Exhale and slowly extend your head forward, elongating the back of your neck and keeping your chin parallel to the floor *(fig. 17a)*.

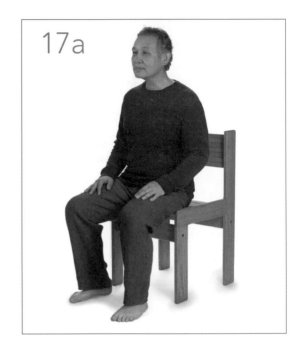

As you inhale, draw your head back to the starting position. With the next exhalation, retract your head, drawing your chin in toward your neck, forcing an extreme double chin *(fig. 17b)*. As you inhale, return to the starting position. Repeat twice more in each direction.

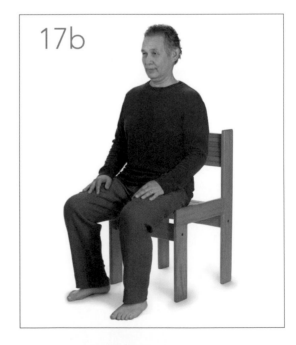

Neck Rolls

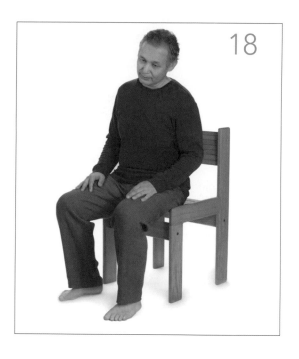

Lengthen your neck. Lower your chin toward your chest and slowly begin to rotate your head in a clockwise direction *(fig. 18)*. Inhale as your right ear crosses over your right shoulder and continue toward the back. Keep the neck extended and long, and do not pinch the vertebral column. Exhale as your left ear crosses over your left shoulder and continue forward. After 3 complete revolutions, reverse and rotate your head in a counterclockwise direction. Try to keep your body relaxed and still throughout, allowing your head to rotate freely.

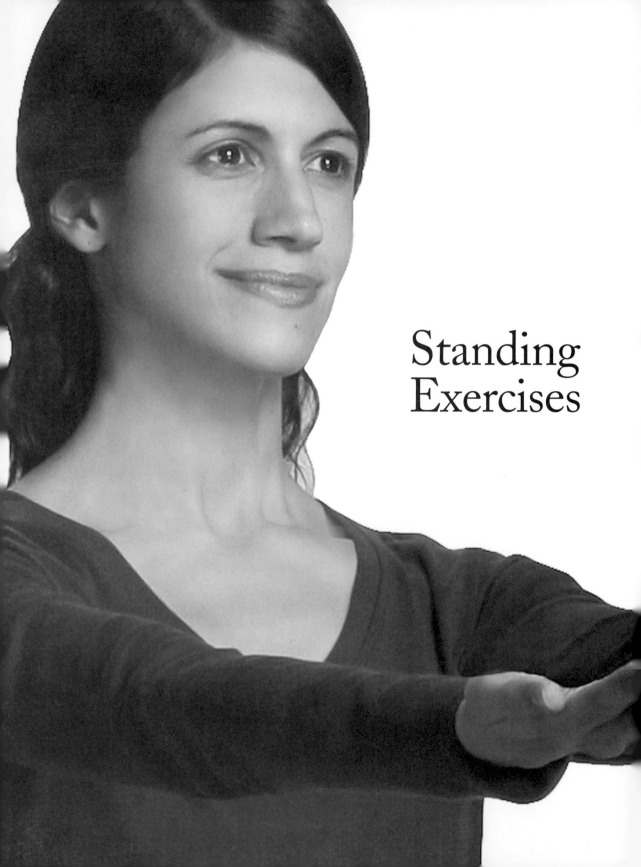

Standing
Exercises

■ Preparation

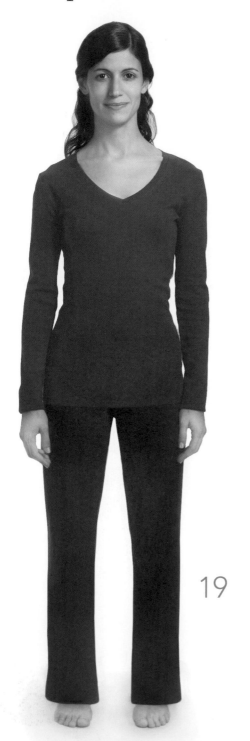

19

Stand on an even surface with your feet parallel and hip width apart. Let the weight of your body rest on the arches of your feet and remain balanced from front to back and side to side. As in the seated posture, elongate through your waist, and slightly elevate your chest. Relax your shoulders, and allow your arms to rest softly at your sides. Elongate the back of your neck and lengthen through the crown of your head. Then soften any rigidity in your body and maintain your alignment with an easy grace *(fig. 19)*.

Take a moment to observe your breathing. Soften the sides of the rib cage and abdomen, and allow the breath to flow smoothly and evenly. Maintain your breath awareness throughout the exercises and as you rest between the poses.

During the following sequence, come back to this simple standing posture after each of the exercises and rest for a moment, being aware of how you feel in your body. Notice each time if and how the exercises have changed how you feel. Unless otherwise indicated, repeat each exercise 3 times, or to your capacity, avoiding strain.

Shoulders ■

Shoulder Shrugs

Keep your head erect and still. As you inhale, slowly raise your left shoulder toward your left ear, contracting the muscles alongside your shoulder and neck *(fig. 20a)*. Hold briefly and then suddenly release the shoulder, dropping it back to its starting position. Repeat with the right shoulder, completing a total of 3 times on each side. Finally, raise both shoulders as high as you can, and hold for several seconds *(fig. 20b)*. Then exhale and slowly lower the shoulders, softening the shoulder muscles completely. Repeat twice more with both shoulders.

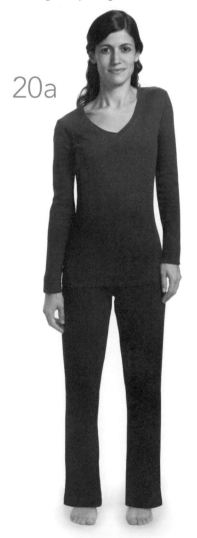
20a

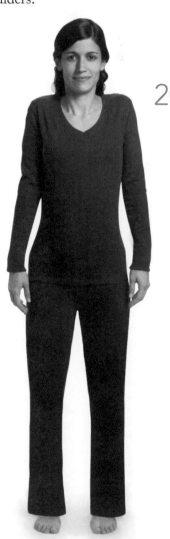
20b

■ Shoulders

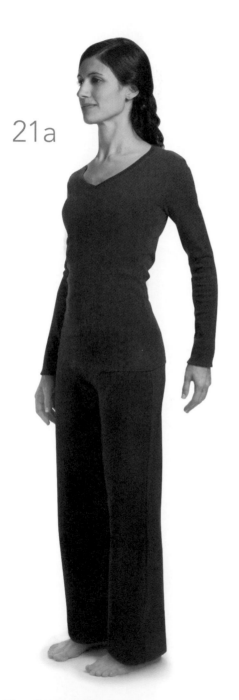

21a

Rotations with Relaxed Arms

Stand with your arms hanging loosely at your sides. Keeping your right shoulder still, exhale and slowly rotate your left shoulder forward. Inhaling, draw the shoulder up toward your left ear, and continuing to inhale, bring the shoulder back as if you are trying to touch the shoulder blade to the spine. Exhaling, lower the shoulder to the starting position, and draw it forward again. Continue circling 3 times, inhaling as you lift the shoulder and draw it back, and exhaling as you lower the shoulder and draw it forward *(fig. 21a)*. Then change direction and repeat 3 more times.

Shoulders

Continue with rotations of the right shoulder, keeping the left shoulder relaxed and still. Finally, rotate both shoulders 3 times in each direction, coordinating the movements with your breath *(fig 21b)*.

While these and the following simple movements require only modest exertion, they are extremely beneficial to the muscles of the shoulder, improving circulation, developing coordination, and expanding the range of movements.

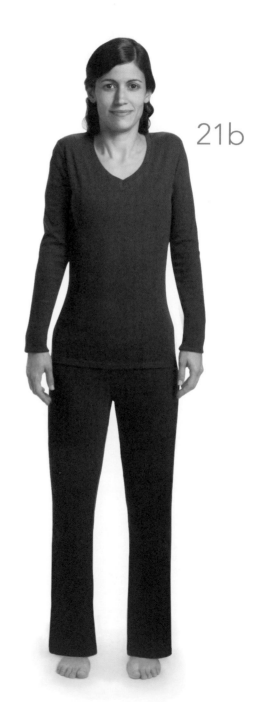

21b

■ Shoulders

Vertical Arm Swings

Make a light fist with both hands, turning your palms to face your body. Keeping your shoulders and arms relaxed, swing your arms forward and back. At first, swing the arms lightly, simply feeling the movement at the shoulder joint. Then begin to involve the shoulders as well. Feel your chest expand as your arms swing back *(fig. 22a)*, and feel your shoulder blades spread apart as the arms swing forward. To increase momentum, bend your elbows on alternate swings *(fig. 22b)*. Continue for 30 seconds or more. This movement is not coordinated with the breath.

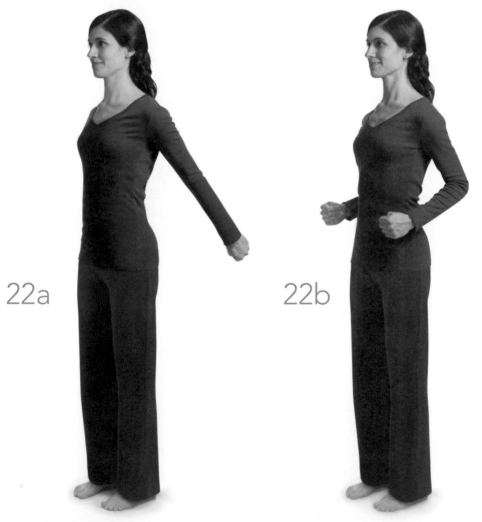

22a   22b

Shoulders ■

Horizontal Arm Swings

Raise your arms to your sides at shoulder height, parallel to the floor, with palms facing down. Keeping your arms straight, begin to swing them forward and back, alternately crossing one arm over the other. Keep your shoulders soft, relaxing any resistance in the pectoral muscles at the front of the shoulders, as well as in the muscles of the upper back.

As your arms swing forward, your shoulders are drawn toward one another in front of your chest and your back expands, separating your shoulder blades *(fig. 23a)*.

As your arms swing back, your chest is expanded, drawing your shoulder blades closer together *(fig. 23b)*. Repeat in a continuous, fluid motion, alternating the arm on top each time. Continue for 30 seconds or more. This movement is not coordinated with the breath.

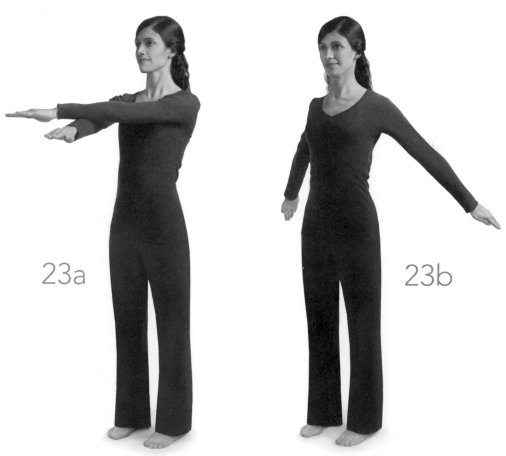

23a 23b

■ Shoulders

Rotations with Extended Arms

Lift your arms in front of you at shoulder level, palms facing up *(fig. 24a)*. Keeping your shoulders relaxed, draw them forward and up, first extending the arms forward and then slowly raising them above the shoulders with palms facing back *(fig. 24b)*. Continue to rotate your shoulders back and down, and as you do, bend your elbows, reach your arms back, and bring your fingertips to your shoulders *(fig. 24c)*. Let the elbows come down in the front until they are about parallel to the floor *(fig. 24d)*. Now reverse direction, raising the elbows, straightening the arms, and reaching the shoulders back

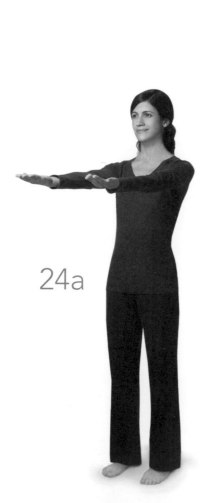

24a

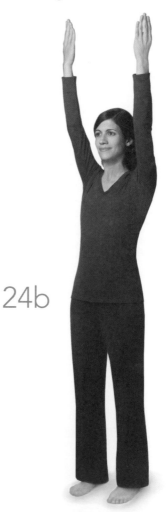

24b

and up. Once the arms are straightened above, complete the forward part of the shoulder rotation and lower the arms, returning to the starting position. Repeat twice more.

Once you are comfortable with the movement, try changing the hand position. Begin with palms facing one another or with palms facing down. Each hand placement will have a different effect on the ball-and-socket joint at the shoulder. You can repeat each variation up to 3 times.

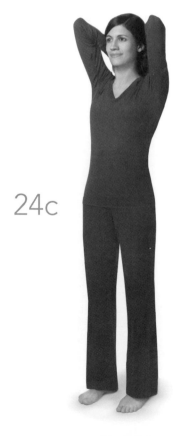

24c

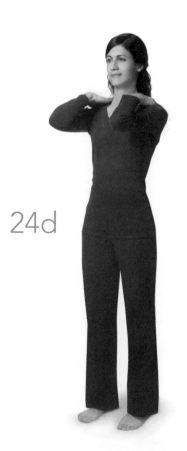

24d

■ Shoulders

Chest Expander

Stand erect. Raise and stretch the arms straight out to the sides at shoulder level, palms facing forward *(fig. 25a)*.

Exhaling, smoothly swing the arms forward, stretching the shoulders forward, expanding the back, and bringing the palms together, fingers lightly touching *(fig. 25b)*.

Inhaling, bend your elbows and bring the palms to the chest. Stretch the chest open, expanding the palms and elbows to the sides without lowering the arms *(fig. 25c)*.

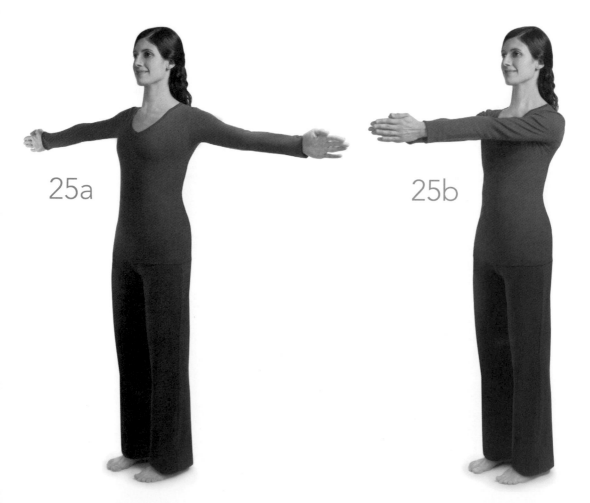

25a

25b

Exhaling, straighten the arms in front once more, stretching the shoulders forward and expanding the back *(fig. 25d)*.

Finally, inhaling, swing the arms open and expand the chest, drawing the shoulders back *(fig. 25a)*.

Repeat the entire sequence of movements 3 or more times, coordinating each movement with your breath.

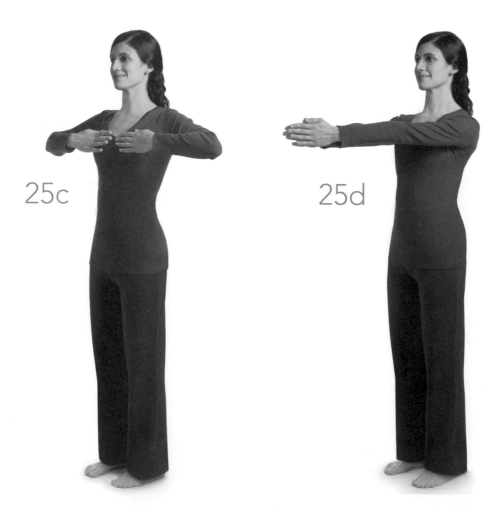

25c

25d

■ Shoulders

Shoulder Wings

Bend your arms and bring your fingertips to the tops of your shoulders, with your elbows facing forward. Press your elbows together, expanding your back and separating the shoulder blades *(fig. 26a)*. Now slowly begin to circle with the elbows as if they were wings. Draw them up in the front *(fig. 26b)*, then circle back, lowering the elbows as the shoulder blades are drawn together. Finally, draw the elbows forward to the starting position. Circle 3 times in each direction.

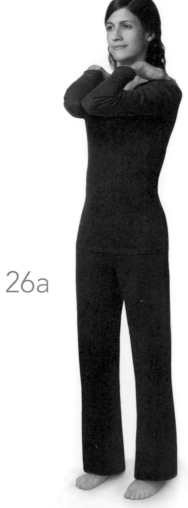

26a

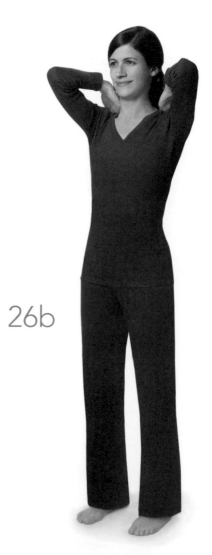

26b

Shoulders ■

Arm Circles

Raise your arms to your sides at shoulder height, parallel to the floor, palms facing down. Keeping your shoulders relaxed and arms straight, circle your arms, starting with small movements and gradually increasing until the circles are as large as possible *(fig. 27)*. Now change direction, continuing with the large circles and gradually decreasing their size until the arms become motionless again. Then lower your arms to the sides and relax.

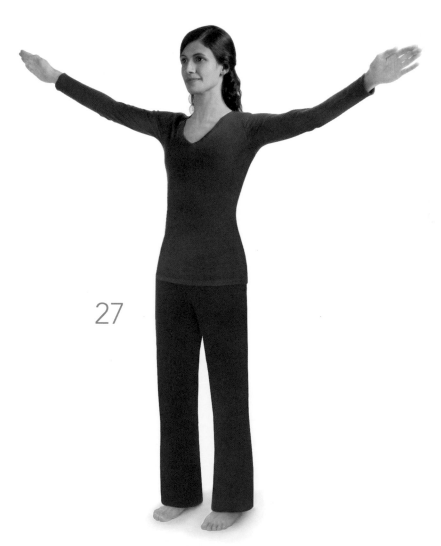

27

■ Hands & Wrists

Wrist Bends

Raise your arms in front of you until they are parallel to the floor. The palms face down with fingers and thumbs together. Keeping your arms and fingers straight, bend at the wrists and raise your fingertips toward the ceiling *(fig. 28a)*. Slowly bring your hands back to the starting position. Then flex the wrists, stretching your hands down with your fingers pointing toward the floor *(fig. 28b)*. Again, slowly bring your hands back to the starting position. Complete 3 repetitions in each direction.

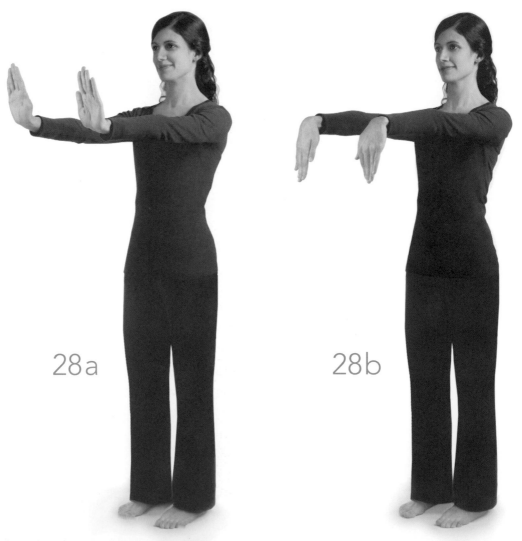

28a   28b

From the original starting position, slowly bend the wrists sideways to the right, pointing your fingers while keeping your palms parallel to the floor. Slowly return your hands to the starting position. Now point the fingers to the left, again keeping the palms parallel to the floor *(fig. 28c)*. Once again, slowly bring the hands back to the starting position. Complete 3 repetitions on each side.

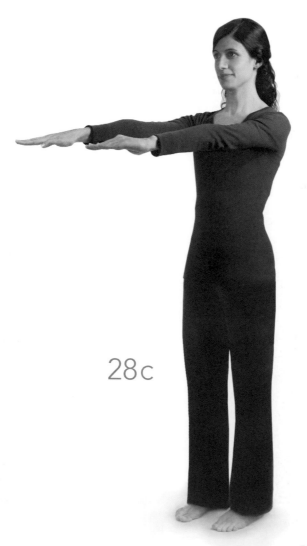

28c

■ Hands & Wrists

Hand Circles

Here are four variations of wrist circling to bring flexibility and strength to your wrist joints.

Begin with your arms raised in front. Bend at the wrists, stretching your hands up with your fingers pointing toward the ceiling. Now with a smooth and fluid motion, circle with both hands, completing 3 full circles, first in a clockwise direction and then in a counterclockwise direction *(fig. 29a)*.

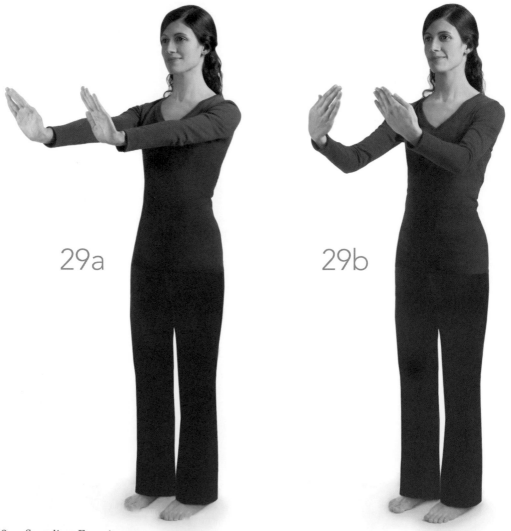

29a   29b

Maintain full extension of the wrists as you circle and try not to let your arms lower toward the floor.

Next, rotate the left hand in a counterclockwise direction while circling the right hand in a clockwise direction. After 3 rotations, change direction and complete 3 more times *(fig. 29b)*.

Now spread the fingers apart as far as possible and circle 3 times in each direction *(fig. 29c)*.

Finally, repeat in both directions with the fingers bent to form tight "claws," fingertips tucked and placed just at the base of the fingers themselves *(fig. 29d)*.

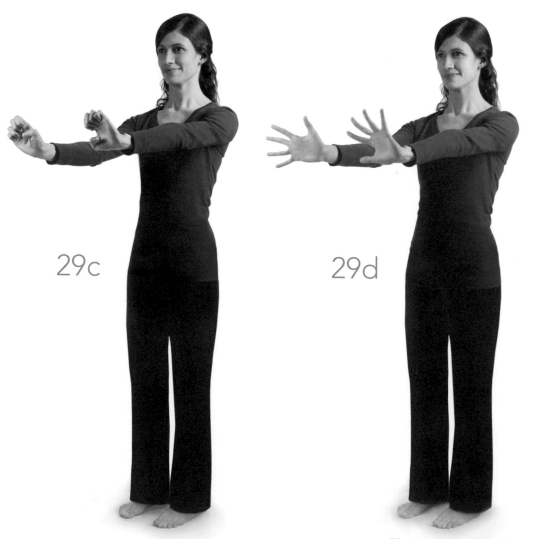

29c   29d

■ Abdomen & Torso

Horizontal Arm Stretch

Raise your arms out to your sides at shoulder height, parallel to the floor. As you inhale, reach through your fingertips as if you are trying to touch the opposite sides of the room *(fig. 30)*. Feel the joints of your shoulders, elbows, wrists, and fingers lengthening. Continue breathing as you hold the stretch. Then, on an exhalation, lower your arms to your sides.

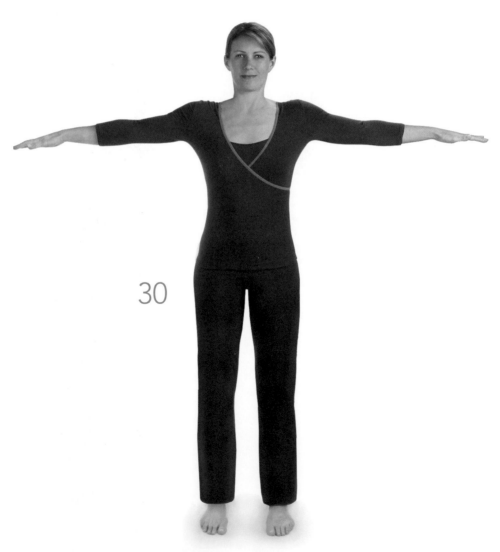

30

Overhead Stretch

As you inhale, sweep your arms out to
the sides and above your head, arms
straight up from your shoulders and
parallel *(fig. 31)*. Keeping your feet
firmly grounded on the floor, stretch up
through your legs and lengthen through
your waist. Slightly elevate your chest
and extend through your shoulders all
the way up through the fingertips.
Simultaneously, draw the head back,
slightly tuck the chin, and lengthen
through the crown of the head. Extend
upward for 2 more inhalations, feeling
as though your entire body is reaching
upward. As you exhale, relax your arms
completely and sweep them slowly back
down to your sides.

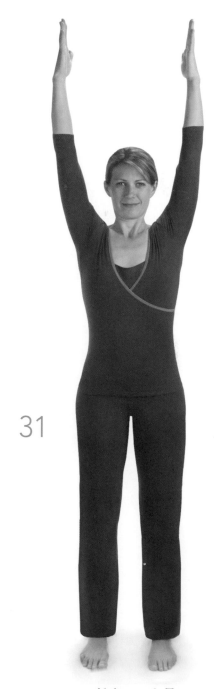

31

■ Abdomen & Torso

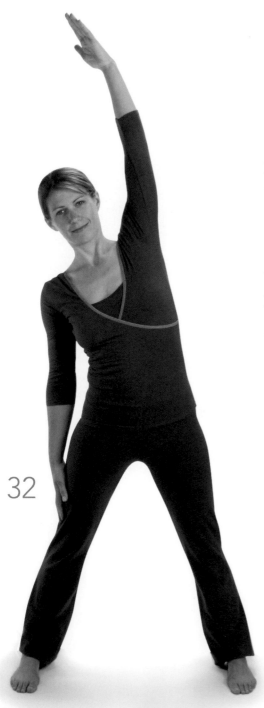

Standing Side Bend

Stand with your feet about 3 feet apart and parallel to each other. As you inhale, sweep your left arm up to shoulder level, then turn your palm up and continue sweeping your arm overhead, bringing it next to your ear. As you exhale, reach up, lengthening the left side of your body, bending slightly to the right. Allow your right hand to slide down your right leg, providing support as you bend *(fig. 32)*. Hold for several breaths, and, as you inhale, bring your torso back to the starting position. As you exhale, lower your left arm to your side. Repeat on the opposite side.

32

Abdomen & Torso ◼

Supported Torso Rotation

With your feet slightly more than hip width apart and parallel to each other, place the heels of your hands on your lower back, fingers spread and pointing down. As you exhale, shift your pelvis forward, supporting your weight with your hands. Now rotate your pelvis to the left, then to the back, and then to the right, making a complete circle *(fig. 33)*. As your hips move, try to keep your head relatively centered. You may find it natural to exhale as you circle forward, and inhale as you circle back. Do a number of repetitions to improve flexibility and coordination. Then repeat in the opposite direction.

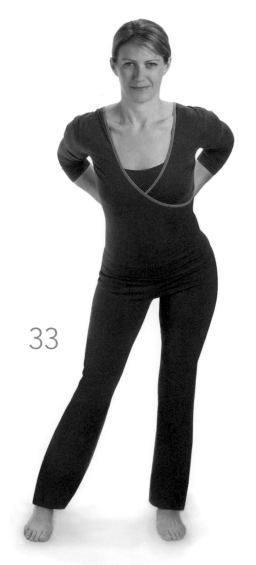

33

■ Abdomen & Torso

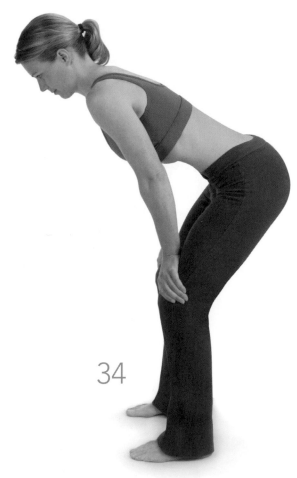

34

Abdominal Squeeze

This important exercise stimulates the circulation of fluids in the abdomen, strengthens the abdominal muscles, and invigorates the abdominal organs. Stand with your feet just wider than hip width and parallel to each other. Bend your knees and lean forward, resting your hands on your thighs with your arms straight. Let the weight of your torso travel down your arms into your hands. Breathe comfortably for a few breaths. Then, as you exhale, firmly contract your abdomen, drawing your navel toward your spine *(fig. 34)*. As you inhale, allow your abdomen to passively relax and expand. Repeat 5 to 10 times.

A variation of the abdominal squeeze is to lower the focal point of the contractions. Instead of focusing on the navel area, focus on the lower abdomen, midway between the navel and the pubic bone. This helps strengthen the muscles of the lower abdomen and improves the tone of the abdominal wall. Again, do 5 to 10 repetitions.

Do not perform the second variation if you have high blood pressure, ulcers, hiatal hernia, or a heart disorder. Women should not perform either exercise during their menstrual period or if pregnant.

Forward Stretch

This exercise is a preparation for all forward-bending exercises. It loosens the hip joints and lengthens the muscles in the backs of the legs and torso.

Stand with your feet well apart and parallel to one another. Inhale and sweep your arms to the sides and overhead, extending your arms from the shoulders, palms facing forward. As you exhale, begin to bend forward from the hip joints, making a circular swimming motion with your arms *(fig. 35)*. Swim forward and down as far as comfortable, and then swim back up.

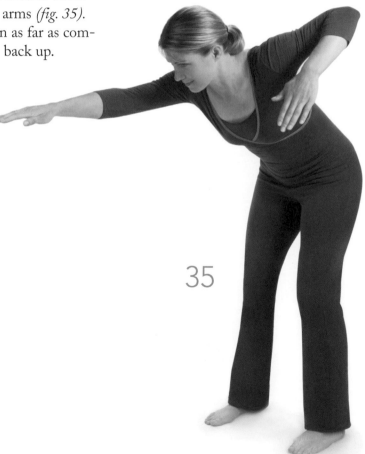

35

■ Legs & Feet

Leg Swings

Stand with your feet parallel and hip width apart. Shift your weight to the right foot and stand tall on the right leg. This will naturally raise your left foot slightly off the floor. Swing your left leg forward and back 10 times, keeping your torso and pelvis steady *(fig. 36a)*. Return to the starting position and repeat the movement on the opposite side.

Once more, shift your weight just enough to the right to maintain balance and raise the left foot slightly off the floor. Next, swing your left leg straight out to the side and then back to the center 10 times, keeping your foot pointed forward and your pelvis level *(fig. 36b)*.

Both these movements will help you improve balance, while the second is a particularly powerful strengthener for the abductor muscles on the sides of the hips.

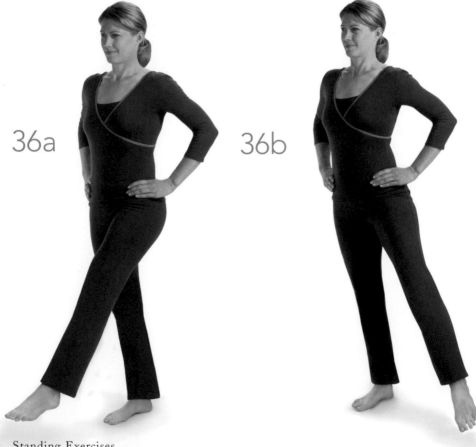

36a   36b

Leg Kicks

This exercise strengthens the hamstring muscles and helps maintain mobility in the knee joints. Stand firm with feet hip width apart. Place your hands at your waist. Shift your weight until it is centered over your right foot. Lift the left foot off the floor and bring it slightly forward. With a sharp movement, kick the left leg back as if to touch the buttocks with the heel *(fig. 37)*. Let the leg return naturally to the starting position and repeat a total of 5 to 10 times. Repeat on the opposite side.

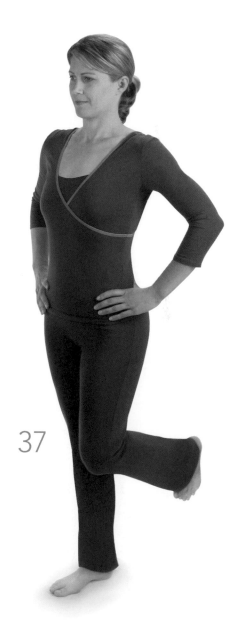

37

■ Legs & Feet

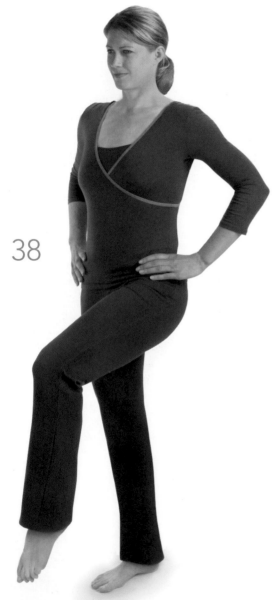

38

Knee Swirls

This movement improves balance and helps maintain mobility and lubrication in the knee joints. With your feet hip width apart, shift your weight to the right, centering your balance over the right foot. Raise your left thigh horizontal to the floor, with your knee bent and your lower leg and foot pointing toward the floor. Circle your foot and lower leg in a clockwise direction, keeping your knee centered *(fig. 38)*. Repeat 3 times, then reverse to a counterclockwise direction. Return to the starting position. Repeat with your right leg.

Dancing Knees

Stand with your feet hip width apart
and parallel to each other. Keep your
weight evenly balanced on both feet.
Tense all the muscles of the left thigh
and around the left kneecap, lifting the
kneecap. Relax and release the kneecap
back down *(fig. 39)*. Alternate with left
and right knees 10 times.

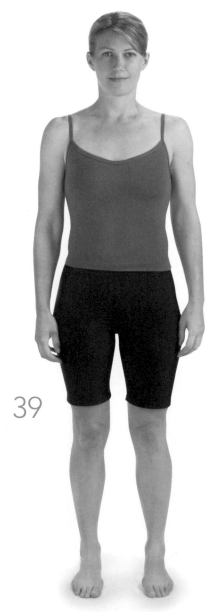

39

■ Legs & Feet

Ankle Exercises

Stand with your feet hip width apart and parallel to each other. Shift your weight over the right leg and lift your left foot off the floor in front of you. You may hold on to a chair or stand near the wall if needed for balance. Flex the left ankle and pull the toes toward you, pointing the toes toward the ceiling *(fig. 40a)*. Relax your foot back to the center. Then slowly flex the ankle in the opposite direction, pointing the toes toward the floor *(fig. 40b)*.

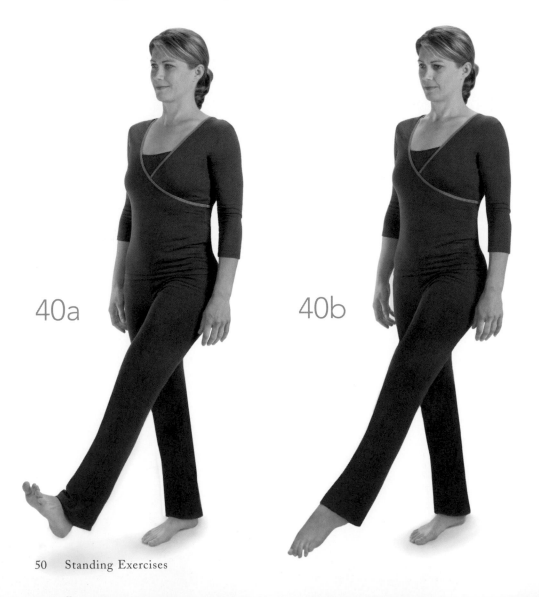

40a

40b

Relax to the center. After 3 repetitions, lower your leg. Repeat on the right side. Again, raise the left foot off the floor. Turn the foot to the left, pointing the toes as far to the left as possible *(fig. 40c)*. Then relax the foot back to the center. Turn the foot to the right, again pointing the toes to the right *(fig. 40d)*. Relax to the center. After 3 repetitions, return to the starting position, and lower your leg. Repeat on the right side.

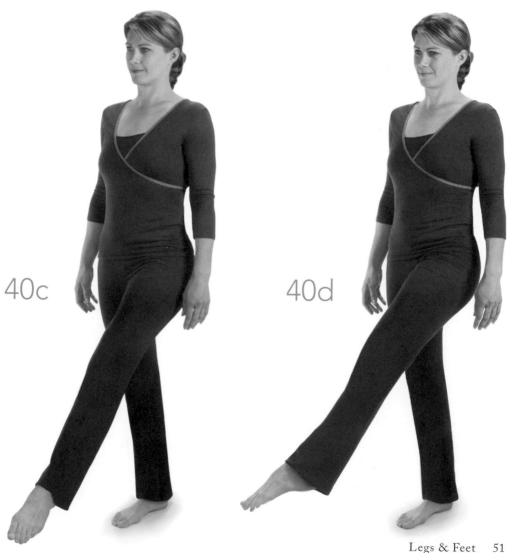

40c

40d

■ Legs & Feet

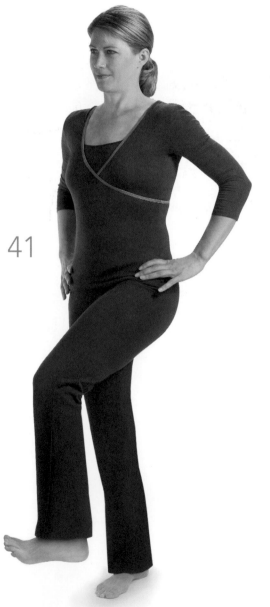

41

Foot Circles

Once again, raise the left foot off the floor and flex it toward you, pointing the toes toward the ceiling. Begin circling at your ankle joint in a clockwise direction. Practice making complete, smooth circles with your foot, with no jerks or pauses *(fig. 41)*. Repeat in a counterclockwise direction. After 3 repetitions in each direction, lower your leg and return to the starting position. Repeat on the right side.

Toe Balance

Stand with your feet together, big toes touching and heels an inch apart. Place your hands on your hips. As you inhale, slowly lift your heels and rise onto your toes *(fig. 42a)*. As you exhale, slowly lower your heels to the floor.

Next, as you inhale, slowly lift your heels and rise onto your toes, holding for up to 30 seconds. Then, slowly lower your heels to the floor once more. For a more challenging exercise, repeat with your eyes closed.

Finally, as you inhale, slowly rise onto your toes while lifting your arms straight in front of you at shoulder level, palms down. Keeping your trunk, arms, and head in line, exhale and slowly turn to the left as far as you can, twisting from the waist and continuing to balance on your toes *(fig. 42b)*. As you inhale, slowly twist back through the center, and exhale as you continue the twist to the right. As you inhale, slowly twist to center and lower your heels and arms to the starting position. For added challenge, repeat one more time with your eyes closed.

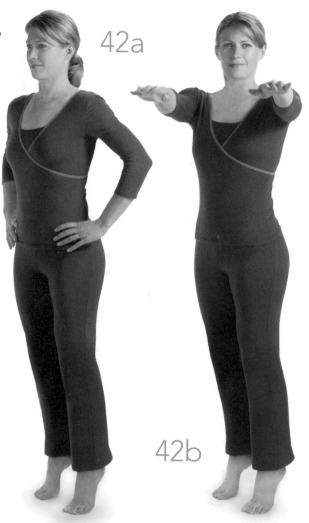

42a

42b

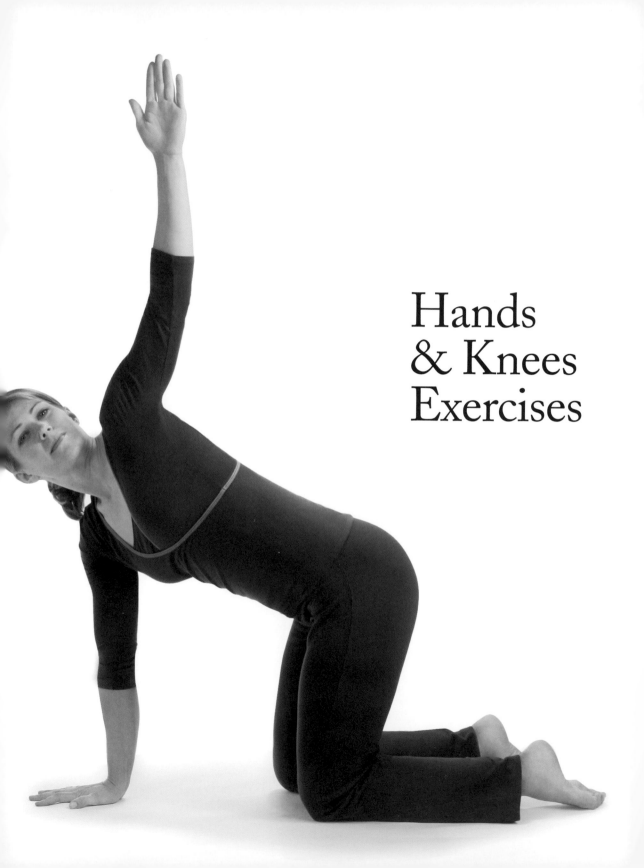

Hands
& Knees
Exercises

■ Preparation

Come down onto your hands and knees (use a mat or blanket for cushioning if needed). Bring your palms directly beneath your shoulders, with your fingers spread as far as comfortable and your middle fingers facing directly forward. Bring your knees directly beneath your hips *(fig. 43)*.

Take a moment before you begin the exercises in the sequence to notice your breath in this posture. Feel your abdomen expand toward the floor when you inhale and contract back toward your spine as you exhale. Allow your breathing to be smooth, deep, and even.

Unless otherwise indicated, practice each exercise only one time, avoiding strain.

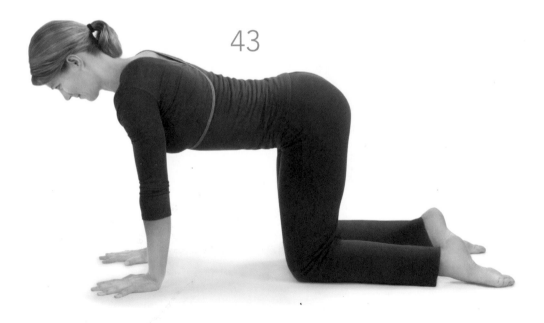

43

Cat Pose

Be on your hands and knees. Exhaling, contract the abdominal muscles, tuck the pelvis, and round the spine, arching the back upward *(fig. 44a)*. Inhaling, release the abdominal muscles as you lift the sit bones, spread the buttocks, lift the head, and arch the spine down. Keep the arms straight and the weight evenly distributed between the hands and knees *(fig. 44b)*. Repeat these movements 5 times.

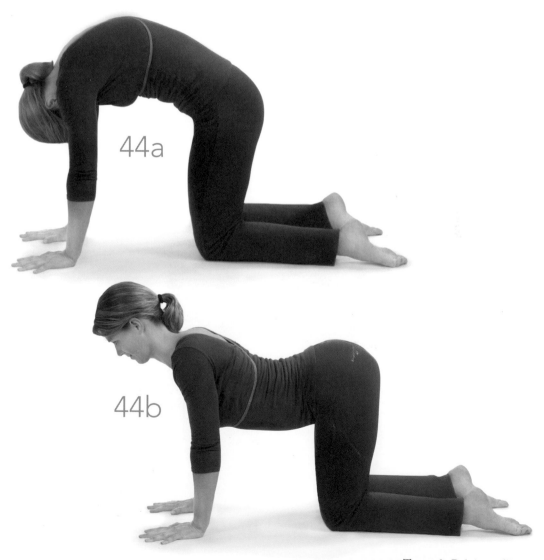

44a

44b

■ Torso & Pelvis

Cat Pose Twist

Bring the palm of your right hand to center, beneath your face. As you exhale, twist to the left, and, keeping your arm straight, sweep it out and up, stacking your left shoulder above your right . Open your chest, reach through the fingertips of your left hand, and turn your head to look up toward your left hand *(fig. 45)*. Hold for up to 5 breaths. As you inhale, lower your arm to the starting position. Repeat on the opposite side.

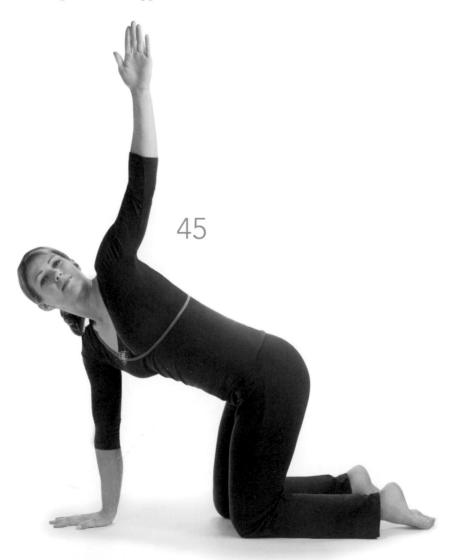

45

Lunge Pose

Step your left foot forward between your hands, your toes in line with your fingers. Extend your right leg straight behind you, resting your knee and the top of your foot on the floor. Keeping your left knee directly above your ankle, shin perpendicular to the floor, lower your pelvis toward the floor, lengthening your thighs in opposite directions, pressing your torso forward, chest lifted, shoulder blades working down your back. Keep your neck long and in line with your spine *(fig. 46)*. If it is not comfortable to have your palms on the floor in this position, come onto your fists or onto blocks. Hold for up to 5 breaths. Repeat on the opposite side.

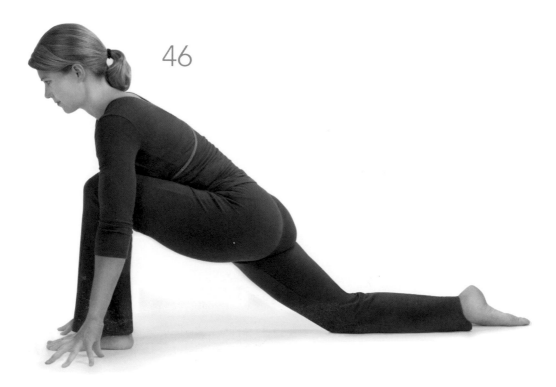

46

■ Torso & Pelvis

Boat Pose

Lie face down on the floor, legs slightly apart, and arms along the body, palms facing your hips. Draw the shoulder blades down your back. Firm your legs and buttocks and press your lower abdomen into the floor as you lift your upper body and legs from the floor, engaging the buttocks and muscles in your lower back *(fig. 47a)*. Keep your legs straight, your arms alongside your body, and the back of the neck long. Hold for up to 5 breaths. As you exhale, release to the floor, turning your head to one side, and rest for up to 5 breaths.

For added strength, repeat with your arms straight out from your shoulders, palms facing down *(fig. 47b)*.

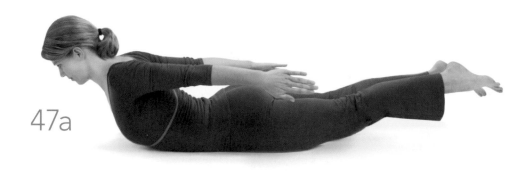

47a

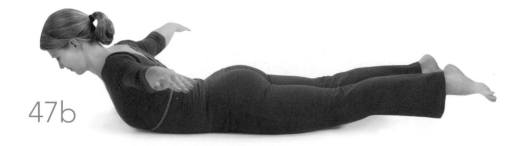

47b

Simple Seated Twist

Sit on a chair or on cushions on the floor. Place the fingertips of your left hand on the chair or the floor near the back of your pelvis, and place your right hand over your left knee or thigh. Keeping your spine erect, gently twist to the left, beginning the twist from your lower abdomen, and then working your way upward to your ribs and shoulders *(fig. 48)*. Follow with your head, looking over your left shoulder. Hold for up to 5 breaths, lengthening your spine as you inhale and deepening the twist as you exhale. Release and repeat on the opposite side.

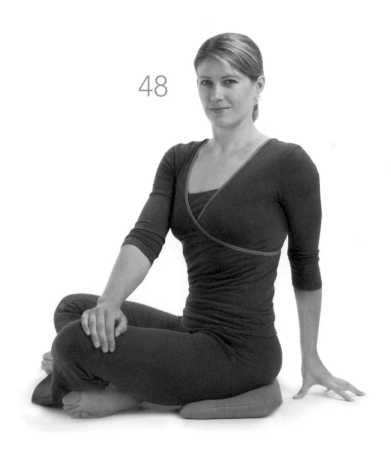

48

Floor
Exercises

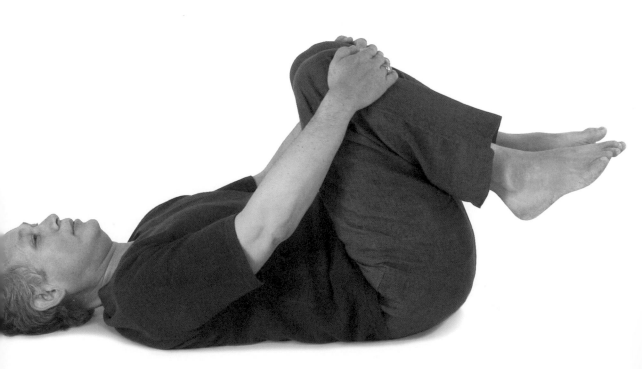

■ Preparation

Lie on your back. Lengthen through your spine and neck. Rest your legs about 6 inches apart, allowing your hips to relax so your feet turn slightly outward. Rest your arms about 6 inches from your sides, palms up. Draw your shoulder blades together and down your back, opening the chest and creating a comfortable surface beneath you on which to rest. Allow your lower back to relax and soften toward the floor *(fig. 49)*.

Notice your breath in this posture. Allow your breathing to become smooth, deep, and even before you begin the exercises.

Come back to this posture after each of the exercises in the floor sequence and rest for a moment, being aware of how you feel in your body. Notice each time if and how the exercises have changed how you feel.

Unless otherwise indicated, practice each exercise only one time, avoiding strain.

49

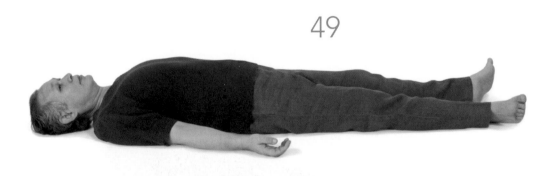

Knees to Chest Pose

Roll your thighs together and point your toes. Bend your left knee and clasp it with your hands, gently drawing your thigh toward your abdomen and releasing your lower back into the floor *(fig. 50a)*. Keep the back of your shoulders, pelvis, and right leg on the floor, and lengthen out through your tailbone. Hold for up to 5 breaths. Release your leg to the starting position, and repeat on the right side. Then, repeat with both knees bent *(fig. 50b)*.

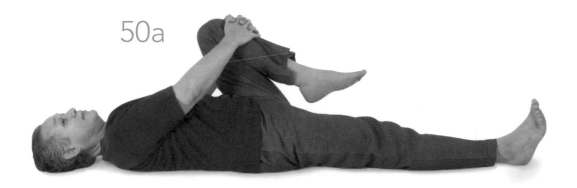

50a

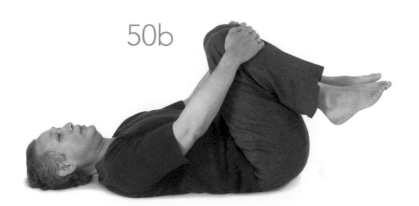

50b

■ Pelvis & Legs

Reclining Leg Cradles

Lying on your back, bend your knees and bring your feet to the floor near your pelvis. Cross your left ankle over your right thigh, and use your left hand against your left thigh to press your knee away *(fig. 51a)*. Hold for 2 to 3 breaths.

Now lift your right thigh toward your abdomen, slide your left arm between your thighs, and interlace the fingers of both hands around your right thigh or shin *(fig. 51b)*. Keep the back of your head, shoulders, and pelvis on the floor. If your head comes away from the floor, support it with a cushion. Soften your face and jaw, and relax through your hips and thighs. Hold for 3 to 5 breaths. To work more deeply into the stretch, gently rock your hips from side to side, drawing your right leg toward your abdomen. Return to the starting position and repeat on the other side.

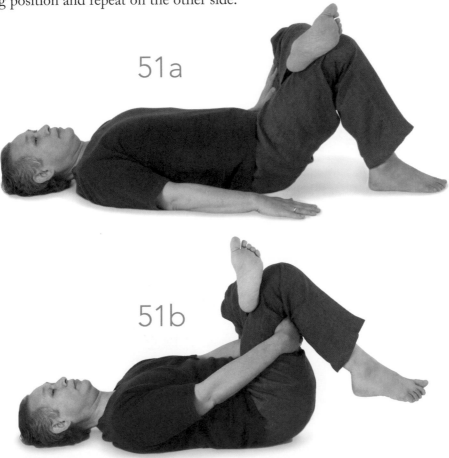

51a

51b

Pelvic Tilt

Lying on your back, bend your knees and bring your feet to the floor near your pelvis, hip width apart, thighs parallel. Bring your arms alongside your torso, palms down. As you exhale, press your lower back into the floor, contracting the abdominal muscles. Then, inhaling, smoothly shift the weight of your lower body to your feet as you slowly lift your spinal column one vertebra at a time. As you raise your torso, lift your abdomen and chest toward the ceiling, keeping the back of your neck long and on the floor *(fig. 52)*. Release as you exhale, lowering from the top of your spine down to the starting position. Inhale and relax. Repeat 5 times.

To work more deeply, come into the spinal arch as before, but lift even higher, drawing your shoulders beneath you, and bringing your breastbone toward your chin. Hold for 3 to 5 breaths. Spread the shoulder blades and then release slowly down the spinal column.

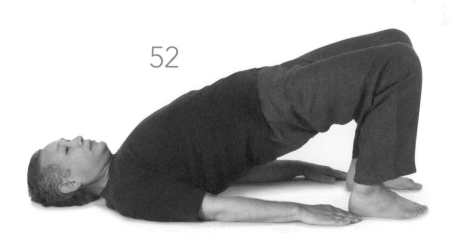

52

■ Systematic Relaxation in Corpse Pose

Relaxation in the corpse pose allows you to integrate and consolidate the benefits of all the exercises in the sequence. It also quiets your mind, restores energy, balances the nervous system, eases strain on the heart, and allows for deep, relaxed breathing.

In this practice, your awareness will move systematically from the head to the toes, and then from the toes back to the head, softening each area of the body, and releasing any tension as you maintain smooth, even, natural breathing.

Lie on your back with your feet about 2 feet apart and your arms alongside your body. If you feel strain in your neck or pressure at the back of your head, you may want to use a thin pillow or cushion to support your head. If you have discomfort in your lower back, place a rolled mat or blanket beneath your knees for support *(fig. 53)*. For warmth, cover yourself with a light blanket, if you wish. Close your eyes and rest, observing the flow of your breath and letting the weight of your body release to the floor. Let the floor support you completely.

Now focus your attention on each of the following areas:

> crown of the head
> forehead and temples
> eyebrows, eyelids, and eyes
> nose *(Hold your attention at the nose for 2 to 4 breaths.)*
> cheeks and jaw
> mouth and chin
> sides and front and back of neck
> hollow of the throat
> tops of shoulders
> upper arms
> elbows
> lower arms
> hands and fingers
> fingertips *(Hold your attention at the fingertips for 2 to 4 breaths, inhaling as if the breath flows down to the fingertips, then exhaling up and out the nostrils.)*
> fingers, hands, and arms

Systematic Relaxation in Corpse Pose ■

shoulders
chest and rib cage, thoracic spine
center of chest, heart and lungs *(Hold attention at the center of the chest for 2 to 4 breaths, inhaling as if the breath flows down to the heart center, exhaling up and out the nostrils.)*
upper abdomen and solar plexus
lower abdomen
sides and lower back
hip joints, buttocks, and inner thighs
thighs
knees
lower legs
ankles
feet
toes and toe tips *(Hold attention at the toe tips for 2 to 4 breaths, inhaling as if the breath flows down into the toes, and exhaling up and out the nostrils.)*

Now bring your awareness to each area in reverse order without pausing for breath awareness.

Finish with 10 or more relaxed breaths, breathing as if the whole body breathes.

To complete your relaxation, gently move your fingers and toes and stretch in whatever way feels good. Then, bend your knees and roll to your left side, supporting your head with your left arm. Rest for up to 5 breaths before sitting up.

53

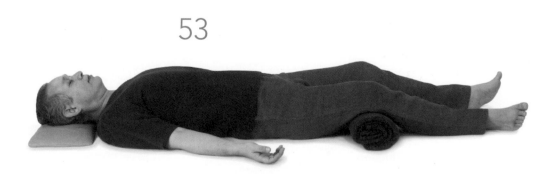

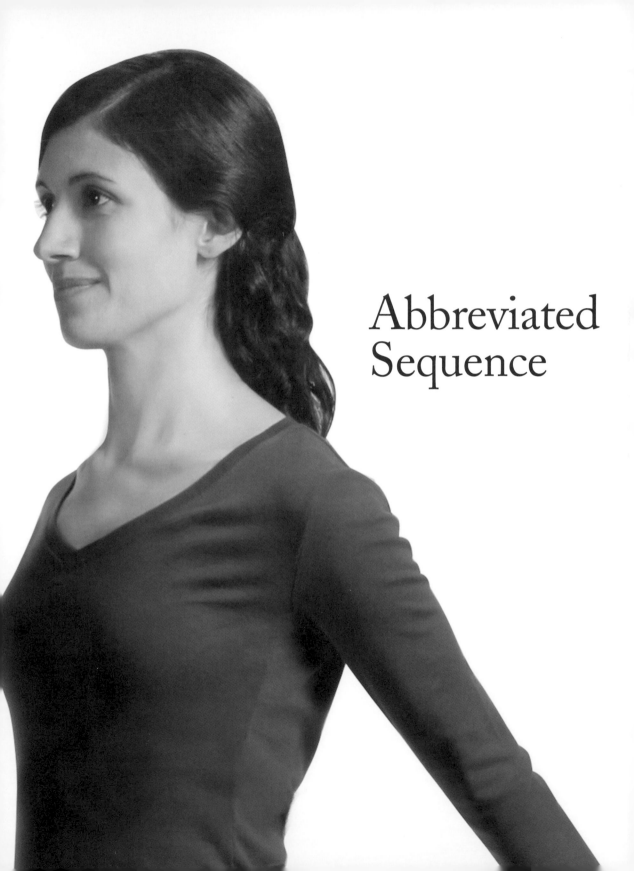

Abbreviated
Sequence

Abbreviated Sequence ■

Even when time is short, just a few minutes of yogic exercises performed regularly can be extremely beneficial. Regularity is the key. The following sequence can be done in fewer than 20 minutes. Use it as a guideline for fitting a regular yoga practice into your life. Experiment with the sequence, substituting different exercises from time to time, and discover what works for you. You may find that on some days you'll want to focus more on the needs of one part of the body than another. Learning to listen to your body's needs is one of yoga's greatest lessons.

■ Seated Exercises

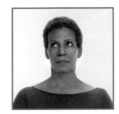
Full-Face Squint

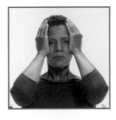
Eye Circles

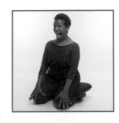
Lion

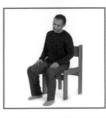
Face Massage

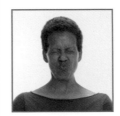
Neck Roll

Abbreviated Sequence

Standing Exercises

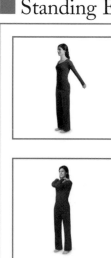 Vertical Arm
Swings

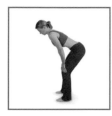 Abdominal
Squeeze

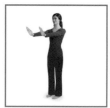 Shoulder Wings

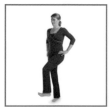 Forward Stretch

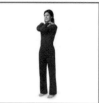 Wrist Circles

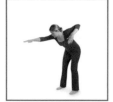 Foot Circles

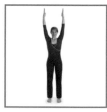 Overhead
Stretch

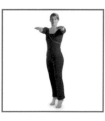 Toe Balance

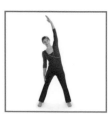 Standing Side
Bend

Abbreviated Sequence ■

■ Hands & Knees Exercises

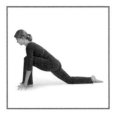
Lunge Pose

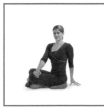
Simple Seated Twist

■ Floor Exercises

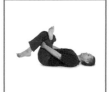
Reclining Leg Cradles

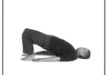
Pelvic Tilt

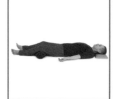
Systematic Relaxation in Corpse Pose

The Himalayan Institute

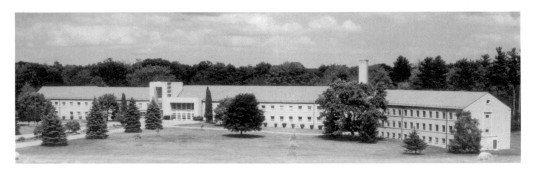

The main building of the Institute headquarters near Honesdale, Pennsylvania

THE HIMALAYAN INSTITUTE OFFERS EDUCATIONAL PROGRAMS, services, and tools for yoga, meditation, spiritual development, and holistic health. The Institute's mission is spirituality in action, and includes a range of global humanitarian projects in addition to its educational activities. Founded in 1971 by Swami Rama of the Himalayas, the Institute draws on its roots in the ancient tradition of the Himalayan masters to facilitate personal growth and development and service to humanity.

Our international headquarters is located on a beautiful 400-acre campus in the rolling hills of the Pocono Mountains of northeastern Pennsylvania. Our spiritually vibrant community and peaceful setting provide the perfect atmosphere for seminars and retreats, residential programs, and holistic health services. Students from all over the world join us to attend diverse programs on subjects such as hatha yoga, meditation, stress reduction, ayurveda, tantra yoga, and yoga philosophy.

The Institute's global humanitarian projects stimulate transformation and social regeneration through a community center model which provides education, health care, and vocational training. As in all of our work, our approach to humanitarian projects is holistic, multidisciplinary, and spiritually grounded.

Programs and Services Include:

- ■ Himalayan Institute Press
- ■ *Yoga + Joyful Living* magazine
- ■ Seminars and Workshops
- ■ Meditation Retreats
- ■ Yoga Teacher Training
- ■ Self-Transformation Program™
- ■ Residential Programs
- ■ Pancha Karma
- ■ Total Health Center and Products
- ■ Spiritual Excursions
- ■ Humanitarian Projects and Community Centers in Africa and India

We invite you to join us. For further information about our programs or humanitarian activities, or to become a member, call 800-822-4547 or 570-253-5551, write to the Himalayan Institute, 952 Bethany Turnpike, Honesdale, PA, 18431, USA, or visit our website at www.HimalayanInstitute.org

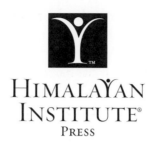

HIMALAYAN
INSTITUTE®
PRESS

THE HIMALAYAN INSTITUTE PRESS has long been regarded as the resource for holistic living. We publish books, CDs and DVDs that offer practical methods for living harmoniously and achieving inner balance. Our approach addresses the whole person—body, mind and spirit—integrating the latest scientific knowledge with ancient healing and self-development techniques. As such, we offer a wide array of titles on physical and psychological health and well-being, spiritual growth through meditation and other yogic practices, as well as translations of yogic scriptures.

Our yoga accessories include the *Chakras: Purifying the Subtle Body* packet for meditation practice and the Neti Pot™, the ideal tool for sinus and allergy sufferers. The Total Health® line of quality herbal extracts is available to enhance balanced health and well-being.

For a free catalog call 800-822-4547 or 570-253-5551
email: hibooks@HimalayanInstitute.org
fax: 570-647-1552
write: Himalayan Institute Press
        952 Bethany Turnpike
        Honesdale, PA, 18431, USA

or visit our website at
        www.HimalayanInstitute.org

Other Resources from the Himalayan Institute Press

Exercises for Joints & Glands DVD
as Taught by Swami Rama
(Available Spring 2008)

Yoga: Mastering the Basics
by Sandra Anderson and Rolf Sovik

Yoga: Mastering the Basics DVD
by Sandra Anderson and Rolf Sovik

Moving Inward: the Journey to Meditation
by Rolf Sovik

Guided Yoga Relaxations CD
Advanced Yoga Relaxations CD
by Rolf Sovik

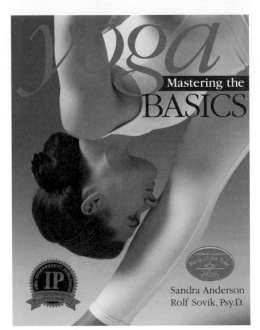

2001 Independent Publisher's Outstanding Book of the Year: Most Life-Changing

Yoga: Mastering the Basics

Sandra Anderson and Rolf Sovik, PsyD

$24.95   B200
Paperback with flaps and lay flat binding
8 1/2" x 11" / 256 pages / 420 duotones

The systematic science of yoga will transform mind, body, and soul. A comprehensive and practical illustrated guide to the essential elements of yoga that cover all aspects of practice: postures, breath-training, relaxation, meditation, and integration of yoga principles into everyday life.

Exquisitely designed with more than 400 high-quality duotones and stunning photography. Included are two 60-minute illustrated posture sequences.

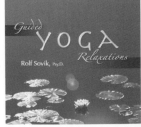

Also available on DVD
$24.95   VDVD0001
Approx. 111 minutes

One convenient DVD provides progressive practice at beginner and intermediate levels. Two guided yoga routines include an introduction and clear, concise instruction by Sandra Anderson.

*Buy both Yoga: Mastering the Basics
book and DVD
for only $35.95 – a 25% savings!*
Item #BDVD 200

Moving Inward
The Journey to Meditation
Rolf Sovik, PsyD

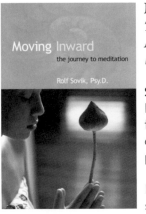

$14.95   B221
Paperback with flaps
6" x 9" / 204 pages

Rolf Sovik shows readers of all levels how to transition from asanas to meditation. Combining practical advice on breathing and relaxation with timeless asana postures, he systematically guides us through the process. This book provides a five-stage plan to basic meditation, step-by-step guidelines for perfecting postures and six methods for training the breath. Both the novice and advanced student will benefit from Sovik's startling insights into the mystery of meditation.

Guided Yoga Relaxations
Rolf Sovik, PsyD

$14.95   CD238
Time 65.15 minutes

Four relaxation and breathing methods will help you soothe anxiety, improve sleep, and reduce stressful thoughts and emotions. In less than 15 minutes you'll feel rested and renewed.